Resurgence 2.

The Quest for Freedom.

Author: Peter. T. Raven.

Yes, my good friends today
say the date

Tue 6 November and I was
going to continue

tell you about further
progress since

the month of September.

Since I last wrote, I've
continued

with my training in the
nursing gymnastics in

Karlskoga two days per week
Mon and

Thursdays with effective
training time on two

And a half hours per day.

My training has mostly been about

balance and strength-building

both legs and arm also some strength training

For the right foot has been included.

But ok, we go into it a little
closer up as we usually do.

Balance training has mostly
been about

stand on one leg at a time,
first the left and

then the right the left leg is no

problems whatsoever.

The right, on the other hand,
have great difficulty

to be able to carry the entire

body weight of itself it is
capable of

Its height just over five to ten
seconds during load.

On balance exercises have
taken place with a

balance disc and it consists of
a round

disc in either wood or plastic
with grooved

pattern so it will not slip,
centered in

the center of its underside a

Ridge that makes when it is in
plant

so are you free from the floor
by using the

your own balance.

This is an art piece in itself
and with

reduced sensation in both
legs and feet make it

all the easier, my biggest
problem, however, is

I miss feel completely in the
heel of the right

Feet and has only little
sensation in the foot's toes.

This affects the outcome, of course, but

I can proudly say that I know

can both stand steadily without falling for

page and can handle even making knee

Bends without losing my balance.

The problem with trying to
get the plate to

Lean first then backward and
from side

to the side is, of course, the
absence of sensation in the

toes and heels I know simply
was not

the foot is and how it is positioned to one hundred

percent.

A further task is the result when

the case of standing balance and its game Console Wii.

With the help of the game and applications

is to keep balance as

for example, go on line is very
difficult

Since you are using your own
body

to balance the figure's slant
on the wire

without falling down, yet
another challenge

available in the game when
you're almost half

Road nothing against you

and you are going to simulate
a jump both feet together

To avoid to fall from the rope.

I can say that this game is not easy to

do even for people with full function but for

us with reduced, it is almost impossible

Although obviously it's a great workout.

No. I did not manage to complete the game.

Well in balance we have also

tried to train up the creek and

Cross back balance and it goes
to like this.

Lying on my back on a wide
bunk with the head on a
pillow now staff hand me

a large rubber ball like thing

though this is a little different
it is more

elongated and a section on
the middle looks

as they tightened the belt
hard at a

large rubber ball.

Well it looks like and lying on
your back

adding up both legs on

increases and should then
with leg

help lift both buttocks and
lumbar so

High as it will go.

This exercise should be
repeated five times

You can keep up.

When it comes to myself so I
can not

lift the right and left sides as
high due to

to the right side is weaker
after stroke

but I can nevertheless, lifting
her ass from

bunk five times and that's
what

The exercise is all about.

An item remains in the
subject balance

training and standing without

fall with the left foot placed
on a round

Plastic ball and this sounds
easy isn't it?

Remember that this is not the
case now remember that

the right leg is difficult to
clear the whole

the body's weight and then
have the fresh

foot on a subject who would
like to roll away.

This is an almost impossible
task

the record for myself is only
five seconds.

Yes, that's what we train in
the balance

In addition to normal walking
without a crutch of course

and to go after a line on the
floor a foot

After the other on the same
route, the same

principle to go on line but
with a

line painted on the floor
instead.

It was balance it.

Strength training then.

We start well with the bone
because it is

What makes the best
progress?

The training has mainly
consisted in

machine training in addition
to balance parts

and have been following.

We have trained leg kick
which means you

sitting in a machine that has
two well stuffed

pillows in front of each leg
and there is a

Substantial weight stacks to
choose from.

Your task now is to press your
legs outwards

to the fully extended position
and then slowly

back with as much weight as
possible and

with both leg help did I just
over

Eighty kilograms in ten
repetitions.

But to make matters more difficult

I was told to use only the right

leg and we started with 10 kg in five

iterations, this went well we are raised to

15 kg and drove five repetitions it

still went well.

I told the staff to increase to twenty

5 kg which they did and it went well

It was getting a bit vibrato with the return

That should be done slowly
and constricting.

We raised to 30 kg and I
passed the five

duplication here but now it
started

receive on both the front and
back movement

and your right knee will be
spasticity at this load.

Oh sorry for those of you who
don't know what spastic

means it is when the leg will
slow up a movement
peacefully but the leg

Instead, the brake releases

repeatedly with no control

that is what is meant by
spastic movement.

After this spastic movement
patterns

I felt now that I wanted to
test how much

weight my right leg actually
managed so

we loaded on 40 kg and I
passed

Still the importance of certain
problems and five repetitions.

This pleased me greatly and
we loaded now

fifty kilograms as resistance I
sat down

grips swaged and as much as I
could

inducing but this heaviness
was simply too

much at least for now.

The next leg is similar

exercise but here you should
press

the legs forward then leg
presses as much

you cope with varying weights

Resistance.

This machine I have tried
before, so

I know that with both leg
force capable

I whole registry with weights,
which means

one hundred forty kg in total,
but this is irrelevant.

What would be tested now it
was right

leg strength and motion
control, so we

started with 20 kg for ten
repetitions and

It went without complaint.

We thus continued with 30 kg
and

nor was that any problem we
increased

further to 40 kg and now it
started

become a hassle for my right
knee that wanted that

usually pump braking on the
way back

Which may not take place?

We decided to increase
further to 50 kg

and it got really heavy for my
right leg

but I pushed myself too clear
the

10 the rehearsal that was the
goal to

The weight would be
approved.

But ok 50 kg is what my leg is
capable of

In leg press right now.

On the strength training have
I tried to

train my right foot by first
working out

with weights and I am
ashamed almost to tell that
right foot only passes a
Resistance on a kg is not a
little bit more.

So instead of weights, we
have tried two

more methods one includes a

rubber string to draw around
your foot in

Height with upper foot pad.

Then, hold against yourself
while you

try to press your feet down
and this is

much harder than it sounds,
and just

This exercise was not
particularly effective

for my part, because my right
foot well

would writhe on the left
under load,

and this led simply to

The rubber band slipped off
my foot.

So a new way to work out the
foot was a

need of physiotherapists had

found an old tool that would

Help me in this work.

The gear is a very simple

construction with two foot
plates with

non-slip, of course, and during
"the pedals

"two pretty heavy duty coil
springs and in

the bottom one wooden plate
to stand firmly on the

the floor.

Therefore, a simple design
that would

Prove to be a real success.

My task is to put both feet on
the

pedals and simply press down
and hold back on the way
back, very simple and very
effective I used to

train with this tool from fifteen minutes up to 30 minutes.

This tool, I recommend hot

To all of you who train out there.

OK wow what I nag haha.

But actually I think it's fun to

write and I share more than
happy with me

of the experiences I had and
what

I itself has benefited greatly
from

Hope you don't mind.

Well what can I tell you more right now?

Well it clearly arms and hand should we not

forget, of course, we have been training them

with.

To begin with, I would like to tell you about what

progress made and how we maintain

Mobility and softness in all
joints.

Firstly, my hand and arm

become stronger muscle wise
and it has

contributed to more mobility
for both arm and

care.

In order to maintain
smoothness and mobility in

my fingers as I sit and bending

soft in a hugging motion and

then slowly, carefully
straighten them completely

I do this on a daily basis
mainly morning and

evening but even on days when I have

While over.

This is good for both to maintain

movement and softness of your finger

results should also be massaging both fingers

and hand and movement but
also for

sense of touch.

Arm and shoulder also need
them

relaxation this is done by

lift both shoulders toward the
ceiling and relaxes

of repeat ten times, the arm
relaxed

by sitting with a table in front
of

themselves.

Stretch out your arm in its
entire length first straight

out and then to the right and
left

page in smooth movements
repeat ten times

Once this is done, leave the
arm of own

power move up toward your
mouth and slowly

Back down repeat ten times.

OK now we're soft and heated
nice

isn't it?

So what has improved since
last time?

In my arm, it has not so much
been

more than that, it has become
a bit more sensitive to

touch and that it gathered
more strength and

can withstand more exercises
without

Slowing as fast as before.

My shoulder still teasing
taunts on

me with hurt and leading
ports a little out

the led on the night which
leads to poor sleep

and of course, pain.

The solution to this concern
believe

physical therapists that it is
mantilla which is

a blue fabric similar band with Velcro

fastening set with one end is made to a

loop and place it over the right arm buttoning

To lie down at the elbow.

Then the rest of the mantilla
be

Over your back against the
left shoulder and over the

another loop is done in this
end with

Velcro mount if you rated it
over

left shoulder you will now put
your right hand in

the loop you created in this
way have your now

arranged a relief for right
shoulder and arm.

I'm told to use the mantilla.

daily and try to follow these

instructions but sometimes
makes it quite

simply to painful to be able to
wear it, but

as I have said, listen always on
staff they

Usually know what is needed.

Over to my right hand.

Changes that have taken
place there is the following.

I can now bend the four out
of five fingers

little finger on the hand did
not want to work

Since day one, it is not much
to say

The more gratifying is that the
thumb index and

middle finger can both bend
over and even

straighten out its own power
which was not

the case in September in
which they could bend

But not straight at all.

Progress thus Similarly, now me

wrist got better than it was in

September it can now bend over both

up and down, but due to the continued

swelling is load still a

Problem.

Some might have been added
in his hand but

not enough to pin and

Keep solid object while I go.

What has been more?

Well I had set up a personal
goal to

able to go one kilometer with
a crutch and it

I hit by far not so long ago

then I decided that being that
take a

walk of just over three and a
half

kilometers.

So this limit I have beaten by
a wide margin would

I probably say.

Without the crutch I would
think that I can handle

Probably five hundred meters
at present.

Indoors I go without a crutch
at all times

But outdoors, it is a must.

As I told you in the previous book so

We carried out a lot of tests regarding

speed from sitting to

turn around, etc.

These tests were done as recently as the first

November 2012 again and I have improved

the results of all tests and this makes

me incredibly happy because it is something

There is no notice under

Training periods.

First November 2012 was also my last

today on sick gymnastics in Karlskoga and

I just want to say a big thank you to all of you

you have been wonderful and
very helpful non mentioned
and non-forgotten.

You know who you are.

My new training camp is now

Orebro University Hospital.

Where did I first day 5
November in

year and what I've seen of it
so far

seems to be very promising
both staff

and also training
opportunities.

My new physical therapist
examined me

carefully so we know which
muscles and joints as

working and which ones need
extra training but some need
training only

To a greater or lesser degree.

My new occupational
therapist has informed me

me about what is to come in

development of the ability and the

both woodwork and kitchen service

means to learn to Cook, bake make coffee etc.

Therefore, such things as are necessary for

To live at home in a normal environment.

The next minor surprise came of her desire me to return the

wheelchair with the comment it needs you No longer since you walk so well.

I thought to myself do I do that?

But in all honesty, she has a great

part right for my wheelchair is
most of the time

still either at home or in the
hospital so

It does no direct benefit for
me.

So in the morning before I go
to Orebro to go in to the
gymnastics and

return it and only keep the
crutch for future support.

This is what can be written
right now

but of course I will come back
again soon

With more news for you.

Today is November 15, 2012
and

Some have occurred since I
last wrote

So we continue will tell.

Since I wrote last, my daily

activities in Karlskoga ceased and

I have moved over to day

rehabilitation in Orebro.

The first thing that happened was that it was

introduced to both staff and with patients and then the usual

Tour.

After introduction, it was time for all

paper with the training schedule and

General information.

My schedule is as follows me

days begin 07.20 then my taxi come to pick

me up for trip to Karlskoga hospital where I

Must wait for service line to Orebro.

For those of you who don't know what Service line

is I can tell you it is a small bus to transport patients between hospitals

Karlskoga and Orebro hospital without fee.

So then a 30-minute wait at

Service line in Karlskoga after the

over to Orebro and the journey takes

approximately 40 minutes to one hour

Depending on how many you want to get

Picked up and what driver it
is.

So at nine time or shortly
thereafter

I tend to be on the site but my
day

do not start until 10.30
o'clock so

There is plenty of time for a
coffee break before

the day begins.

 This particular gap, I have
talked to

the staff and I will probably

Start at 10 in the future.

Well my day begins at present

with a pass physical therapy
followed by a

Pass with occupational
therapy since lunch

followed by another then

physical therapy and
occupational therapy which

End my day at 14.30 hours.

Service line is home to 15:00
and I am

at the hospital in Karlskoga at
approximately

16:00 time and my
connection taxi

home will not until 16.40 so
unfortunately

much of my time goes away in
travel time and

At home, I am home at 17 and
trust me then you are
completely finished.

Oh good back to training and work therapy in Orebro.

Firstly, I would like to mention that I'm not

use the wheelchair further and the decision was made together with the therapy and physiotherapy.

How it goes?

Well actually really good leg becomes

stronger and stronger day by day and

I'm out and walking about three

kilometers per day whether I'm

Free or not.

So for those of you out there who are struggling and it

seems pointless never stop fighting

each thing you do will help much more than

you believe and you will
succeed if you

set small goals all the time I
know

I did it myself.

So my only companion on the
road

Now is Mr. crutch and we will
continue the path together
and has worked

Very well so far but.

Unfortunately, it will be
replaced next

week towards a more modern
red with

soft ergonomic handle.

I have also submitted the application for

both the disability allowance and car allowance

and now await only a medical certificate to

Add and precisely it can be

difficult to obtain but shock on the whole

Time to give those with him.

Yes, I have tried to drive a car
already

and it runs really good but the
one that I

going to buy must get some
reconstruction

for the problem with my right
hand and arm.

The problems in the right arm
and the hand is probably
caused by an injury

which I do not remember that
I done to me but according to
the doctor, it is something
broken.

So this Friday November 16

starting my day with an x-ray
and a

meeting with the surgeon.

The same day, I have a
scheduled

meeting with the hospital's
neurons psychologist

who wants to talk to me for
two hours so

my morning workout
disappears completely

but I've still have my own

Afternoon sessions as luck
would have it.

Training sessions consists of
the following torque.

First I'm starting my pass with
five

minute warm-up on training

cycle with 1, 5 kgp resistance and may

using the staff to bind fixed me

right hand on the handlebars and my right foot at pedal.

This is because the hand is not strong

enough to hold on to the handlebars and foot

turning toward the crankset.

Yes, we continue to the next station and

This is to work out the right arm with

using a device attached to a bench

and weights I'll explain.

It takes place on the bench
and places

right arm in something that
looks like a

long Crescent formed support
for arm

and at the end a grip handle,

the handle is sitting on a
position that is

adjustable for best
adaptation.

At the front there is a loop
that moves weights

can be attached and in my
case only one kilo

for the time being.

It takes place on the bench
and put

arm in support and grip the handle

but I get the same way tight fast my hand around the handle bar to be able to work out at all.

Staff will help me with it and also

To hook in weight on the handle.

We must now bring his hand
and

the arm that working towards
the body so

many times as possible and it
is

tall order despite the low
weight but

the hardcover and shoulder does still hurt but the exercise must

implemented for training's sake and for

Continued movement of the arm.

The following station is the leg press.

This machine is a construction man

step into and grips and

at the front there is a large
foot plate of

aluminum which is attached
to a

adjustable weight stacks.

My exercise to gouge both

legs to almost fully extended
mode

with a weight resistance on 40 kg and

This is repeated 30 times for my part.

Now over to the bar and sitting

training.

Lying on your back should I now raise both

arms over head as far as it will
go without doing pain and it
can be a bit tricky given sore
arm and shoulder.

But this should be done in my
case 2 x 10 times and it is a
huge effort but necessary for

The bodies further operation.

Now in a sitting position, I will now take

up your shoulders towards your ears and then

slowly lower them down again and this

Repeat 2 x 10 times.

Further exercises in prone
position Is the following.

Laying on back bend both legs
and

put them down in the couch
when you have bent

knees and from this location
you should now

fold one leg to the side while you

hold the other stable in bunk

Repeat 2 x 10 times each leg.

We continue with the pelvic lift.

Lying on your back, you should now

Lift

the tail from bunk and lower slowly

back this operation is repeated 2 x 10

times.

Another exercise while lying on the back.

To now trail the entire leg to the side

your toes should point toward
the ceiling all the time

And the leg should not be
lifted from the couch.

This step is repeated 3 x 5
times.

The training session ends with
a

Seated exercise and it is as
follows.

Add up the right leg in its
entire length

on the couch and fall
forwards in

the hip until the strain is felt
in the back

thigh hold about 30 seconds
and

then do the same with the

left leg.

You will see my workouts three days

per week but note that two days

This week is the twin such that.

Sure it's tough and very

frustrating but if you that I
own

the stubbornness, it will

very well to use during this

training.

OK moving on to occupational
therapy.

Yes, for one, starts working
therapy

to sit at a table with a

towel under my arm and
working

forward and to the sides
about five to

Ten minutes to loosen up
your joints.

Since I usually use me by

a soft tag ball to stimulate

The nerves of the hand and arm.

Now we're going to try to do something specific

of it all.

At the time of writing I have not had time

try on so much yet but I have

tried to get up and place

around Styrofoam ball and
place them on

A Board with the intended
hole.

The most recent result was 20
balls in

various sizes placed and
removed

Picked which is a good result.

Then I tried to unscrew the

a plastic nut from a plastic screw

worse results because the hand does not

Capable of turning just squeezing.

I should add that I have big problem

with movement in my hand
because of

Swelling and poor blood
circulation.

This will be checked up on
Friday 16th

November and I hope of
course that

It is possible to solve in any
way regardless of

If it means surgery.

So my training in the field of occupational therapy is

limited but the balls, I will

continue with because it trains both

grip and release movement of the hand and the

More training, the stronger it becomes.

This pass is run twice daily
two

times a week and I have
pretty high hopes for myself.

Well this is what I can write
just now but I will be back a
little later

with more information about
what

happening and what is
planned ahead

for one, both in terms of
training and

occupational therapy and also

insurance I will keep you

Informed I promise.

Friday 16 November. Yes,
today has the

been full speed but not quite what I

expected by day.

I found myself at the hospital at about

09.15 and made it with a cup of coffee

then I was told by the nurse

that right after lunch I would at

x-rays of my hand and wrist at

because of the swelling and pain from

hand and wrist.

But first, I have an appointment with the neuron

psychologist between 10 and 12 and his

Job is the following.

He picked up various drawings

I would copy to see how well

the brain is capable of this

the task, then rattled off a

list of words and you'll repeat
the

He speaks the words he read
15 words

and I was able to reproduce
the five or six

pieces.

This list was read up about five

times and I could remember

about five or six words each

time, then, he read up further

a list of 15 words and the result was

like, in conclusion, he read up

all words with a new involved
and

I would render the words I
recognized

and say in which of the first
two

lists they were or if they were
not there

with at all, and which I
managed to better

Would think about 15 words
properly positioned.

More information was to
delete numbers from

a mixture of numbers and to
follow

lines between bullets and
numbers, and

do I need to add that it was
time to

All test.

This was what we had time on
our two

hours.

A new meeting with him is scheduled

on Monday next week for further

tests and there will also be a

third meeting focusing on car

Run time.

OK now we take lunch!

The time now is 12:30 pm and
I'm on my way

for emergency Radiology
reception and well

in place so it was my hand
carefully

studied and they quickly saw
that it was

abnormally swollen and
fingers and

wrist hard to bend.

So they x-rayed first hand
with

fingers from both above and
in

side to side then came wrist
from above

and from the side since I was asked

To wait in the waiting room at the result.

The nurse came a bit later and

explained to me that the result had

sent directly to my doctor by computer

And I could go back to the
rehabilitation.

So I had to take the crutch
and

wander back to the Division
where

the nurse met me and told
me I

have time for some therapy before

ends for the day.

OK then, only to wander away to

Nursing gymnastics then met me

physical therapist myself and we started

with a bit of arm bends into
the machine I

described in the past but I can
not

many because of pain in the
arm

and shoulder.

Well she thought we skip the
arm and

walking on the leg press
instead and I

drove my 30 repetitions on 40
kg

then I said that I wanted to
feel on the

the weight of 50 kg and did
even 10

repetitions with the weight.

So will continue the weight of

Leg press be 50 kg nothing else.

We went to the bench for exercise

that is to lie on your back with

knees bent and one leg to the side

While the other stays stable.

This is repeated ten times
each leg and

There were no major
problems then became

I asked to put me up on

the edge of the bench with
your feet on the floor.

My physical therapist then mounted a

ten-kg weight on my right leg and asked

me extend it fully and repeat

torque 10 times which I

Managed.

Good, she said, and placed
more

a ten-kg weight on my left leg
now

We go every two legs starting
with the left

running ten then switch to the
right and run

Ten repetitions which I did.

She asked if I tried to be

on your toes? I answered no
because I

had not tested this item so we

went to the barren and there I
had to go up

on your toes 10 times very
good, she said it

may suffice for today.

After this hectic day, it
became

journey home again at 15 and
one hour

While waiting for the
connection taxi to

come all the way home so we
may ensure

week what is going on, we
heard then.

OK here we go since then has
the following occurred.

Last Monday the 19/11 got

I granted the hospital
journeys by private taxi

because no taxi was booked
on me.

morning with the result that I

missed the service line.

On Wednesday it was training
in normal

courses with a little extra in
the morning

because I start at 10 instead

Ten and thirty.

But then last Thursday came a
heavy

notice we were asked to
immediately travel

to Uppsala to our mother's
cancer

had become much worse, so
we did

us ready and went by car
there.

I and my siblings sat on the
wake of

our mother almost 24 hours a
day so

very little sleep there was and
our dear

mother fought in the last days
to be

here, but on Saturday 24/11
2012 found

She finally peace and she is
very

missed by us all.

Rest in peace beloved mom.

I will of course continue me

training and my struggle to get

back but this event will

of course, to reflect in me

continuing struggle.
 My priority right now is to find a

home ownership because in
these times

pass neither I nor my siblings
to

be around each other we all
need peace

and quiet and that is why it is
a must to

arrange your own
accommodation at any time
during the

next week.

So dear readers I will return
later

with more information about
what

happening around me and of
course I'll

mention when this was
written today is the

Sunday 25/11 2012.

Yes, today is 27/11 2012 and
it

 has not been so much more
about

training I have done 6 minutes

walking test which means you
go in a

corridor which is 25 meters
long back and

back as many times as you
want on

six minutes.

My case I managed to go six
rounds, then,

300 meters around then I had
to

stop because I was tired and

balance bad and my right foot

drops and get stuck in the
floor which

Risk stumbling and falling.

After the test, we agreed that

My foot contraption do I use
the full

time and I need to practice
my thighs

muscles a lot we tried even to

get up on your toes which
goes with great

difficulty.

As you probably understand,
it is difficult

to find your desire in the
present

circumstances so I will for this

Time to tell a little joyful
news.

My efforts to get the drive
again

seems to be coming true body

wise, I have the strength and
the application is

submitted to the social
insurance office if

car allowance and the only document I

need is the physician's assessment and

the I will require tomorrow then

I just need to wait for the decision of the

the social Insurance Agency.

So, with these words I end this

Part 2 of the return but a

final part Will OF Course

commence as soon as
possible because the series
will

Follow me for a year.

I wish you all a very Merry
Christmas

And a happy new year 2013.

Of course, a huge thank you
for caring

staff and wards in the
relevant parts.

I hope we can hear about it in
my third and final writing on
the return from a stroke big
hug to all of you out there and
you remember never stop
fighting and good luck.

See you in 2013.

With a warm greeting

P. Raven.